healtnier you

FOOD JOURNAL+

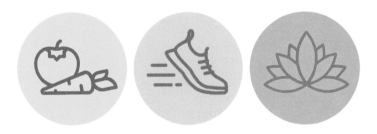

90-DAY NUTRITION, FITNESS, AND WELLNESS TRACKER

ROCKRIDGE PRESS

> >

Using This Journal

If you're reading this, congratulations! You're already one step closer to your goal. Whatever that goal may be—confidence, energy, overall health—this journal can be a powerful tool in making it happen. Recording your choices and feelings around your health on a daily basis not only makes you more accountable to yourself but also helps you become more aware of your patterns in general. Seeing your weekly progress helps you stay motivated. No matter where you're coming from or what your goal is, this journal will be by your side during the journey.

Tips

Be detailed about tracking. Don't forget to record the small bites in between meals or the four flights of stairs you climbed to the doctor's office.

Tailor the daily entries to your needs. Want to record your weight daily? Write it in the margin. Intermittent fasting? Use one of the meal sections to note the hours of your fast. Having a hard time with cravings? Write them down under "How I Felt About Today" or "Additional Notes."

Take advantage of the "Additional Notes" section. Whether it's your daily multivitamin, a new habit, or a simple act of self-care (such as finally making that doctor's appointment or finding time to meditate), the more details you can track about how you're taking care of yourself, the better.

15 Suggestions for Healthy Habits

1. Start and end your day with a thought of gratitude.

2. Aim to get two or three servings of vegetables each day.

3. Plan your meals for the week.

4. Limit your screen time by turning off your phone notifications and turning off the TV one hour before going to sleep.

5. Spend 10 minutes stretching to some relaxing music in the morning.

6. Take a walk after dinner, even if it's just around the block.

7. Tidy up an area of your living space for 10 minutes every day.

8. Practice eating slower. Enjoy every bite rather than rushing through a meal.

9. Do an activity that makes you happy, like dancing or gardening.

10. Meditate each day to improve your mindfulness.

11. Start lifting weights. You'll feel powerful!

12. Keep healthy snacks in the house for energy emergencies.

13. Do something creative or mentally stimulating every day.

14. Replace unhealthy habits (sugary treats, smoking) with healthy ones (going for a walk, calling a friend).

15. Don't restrict yourself from enjoying life, but don't be afraid to set necessary boundaries.

My Goals

What is your main goal for the next 90 days?

....
....
....
....
....

Do you have other goals, as well?

....
....
....
....
....

What are your biggest challenges? Strengths?

....
....
....
....

How are you feeling about getting started?

....
....
....
....
....

My Starting Point

Date: ....

Circle the level you're at in the following areas, then elaborate further on the following lines.

(1 = poor, 2 = needs work, 3 = okay, 4 = good, 5 = excellent)

Diet   1   2   3   4   5

....

....

....

....

....

....

Exercise   1   2   3   4   5

....

....

....

....

....

Sleep   1   2   3   4   5

....

....

....

....

....

....

Stress   1   2   3   4   5

....
....
....
....
....

Confidence   1   2   3   4   5

....
....
....
....
....

Energy   1   2   3   4   5

....
....
....
....
....

Are there any other measurements you'd like to track?

....
....
....
....
....
....
....
....

DAYS
1–30

>>

DATE _____ SLEEP _____ HOURS

QUALITY OF SLEEP ○ POOR   ○ ADEQUATE   ○ GOOD

MEAL 1	SNACKS / BEVERAGES
MEAL 2	
MEAL 3	

HYDRATION ◇ ◇ ◇ ◇ ◇ ◇ ◇ ◇

ACTIVITY	DURATION	NOTES

MOOD	MORNING	AFTERNOON	EVENING

HOW I FELT ABOUT TODAY	ADDITIONAL NOTES

DATE.. SLEEP............ HOURS

QUALITY OF SLEEP ○ POOR ○ ADEQUATE ○ GOOD

MEAL 1	SNACKS / BEVERAGES
MEAL 2	
MEAL 3	

HYDRATION ◇ ◇ ◇ ◇ ◇ ◇ ◇ ◇

ACTIVITY	DURATION	NOTES

MOOD	MORNING	AFTERNOON	EVENING

HOW I FELT ABOUT TODAY	ADDITIONAL NOTES

DATE... SLEEP.................HOURS

QUALITY OF SLEEP   ◯ POOR   ◯ ADEQUATE   ◯ GOOD

MEAL 1	SNACKS / BEVERAGES
MEAL 2	
MEAL 3	

HYDRATION   ◇   ◇   ◇   ◇   ◇   ◇   ◇   ◇

ACTIVITY	DURATION	NOTES

MOOD	MORNING	AFTERNOON	EVENING

HOW I FELT ABOUT TODAY	ADDITIONAL NOTES

DATE.. SLEEP................HOURS

QUALITY OF SLEEP   ◯ POOR   ◯ ADEQUATE   ◯ GOOD

MEAL 1	SNACKS / BEVERAGES
MEAL 2	
MEAL 3	

HYDRATION   ◇ ◇ ◇ ◇ ◇ ◇ ◇ ◇

ACTIVITY	DURATION	NOTES

MOOD	MORNING	AFTERNOON	EVENING
HOW I FELT ABOUT TODAY	ADDITIONAL NOTES		

DATE_____ SLEEP_____HOURS

QUALITY OF SLEEP   ○ POOR   ○ ADEQUATE   ○ GOOD

MEAL 1	SNACKS / BEVERAGES
MEAL 2	
MEAL 3	

HYDRATION   ◇   ◇   ◇   ◇   ◇   ◇   ◇   ◇

ACTIVITY	DURATION	NOTES

MOOD	MORNING	AFTERNOON	EVENING

HOW I FELT ABOUT TODAY	ADDITIONAL NOTES

DATE.. SLEEP............HOURS

QUALITY OF SLEEP ○ POOR ○ ADEQUATE ○ GOOD

MEAL 1	SNACKS / BEVERAGES
MEAL 2	
MEAL 3	

HYDRATION ◇ ◇ ◇ ◇ ◇ ◇ ◇ ◇

ACTIVITY	DURATION	NOTES

MOOD	MORNING	AFTERNOON	EVENING

HOW I FELT ABOUT TODAY	ADDITIONAL NOTES

DATE.. SLEEP.................HOURS

QUALITY OF SLEEP   ◯ POOR   ◯ ADEQUATE   ◯ GOOD

MEAL 1	SNACKS / BEVERAGES
MEAL 2	
MEAL 3	

HYDRATION ◇ ◇ ◇ ◇ ◇ ◇ ◇ ◇

ACTIVITY	DURATION	NOTES

MOOD	MORNING	AFTERNOON	EVENING

HOW I FELT ABOUT TODAY	ADDITIONAL NOTES

DATE.. SLEEP............HOURS

QUALITY OF SLEEP ○ POOR ○ ADEQUATE ○ GOOD

MEAL 1	SNACKS / BEVERAGES
MEAL 2	
MEAL 3	

HYDRATION ◇ ◇ ◇ ◇ ◇ ◇ ◇ ◇

ACTIVITY	DURATION	NOTES

MOOD	MORNING	AFTERNOON	EVENING

HOW I FELT ABOUT TODAY	ADDITIONAL NOTES

DATE.. SLEEP.............HOURS

QUALITY OF SLEEP   ○ POOR   ○ ADEQUATE   ○ GOOD

MEAL 1	SNACKS / BEVERAGES
MEAL 2	
MEAL 3	

HYDRATION   ◇   ◇   ◇   ◇   ◇   ◇   ◇   ◇

ACTIVITY	DURATION	NOTES

MOOD	MORNING	AFTERNOON	EVENING

HOW I FELT ABOUT TODAY	ADDITIONAL NOTES

DATE.. SLEEP...............HOURS

QUALITY OF SLEEP ○ POOR ○ ADEQUATE ○ GOOD

MEAL 1	SNACKS / BEVERAGES
MEAL 2	
MEAL 3	

HYDRATION ◇ ◇ ◇ ◇ ◇ ◇ ◇ ◇

ACTIVITY	DURATION	NOTES

MOOD	MORNING	AFTERNOON	EVENING

HOW I FELT ABOUT TODAY	ADDITIONAL NOTES

DATE.. SLEEP............HOURS

QUALITY OF SLEEP   ○ POOR   ○ ADEQUATE   ○ GOOD

MEAL 1	SNACKS / BEVERAGES
MEAL 2	
MEAL 3	

HYDRATION   ◇ ◇ ◇ ◇ ◇ ◇ ◇ ◇

ACTIVITY	DURATION	NOTES

MOOD	MORNING	AFTERNOON	EVENING

HOW I FELT ABOUT TODAY	ADDITIONAL NOTES

DATE.. SLEEP............HOURS

QUALITY OF SLEEP   ⃝ POOR   ⃝ ADEQUATE   ⃝ GOOD

MEAL 1	SNACKS / BEVERAGES
MEAL 2	
MEAL 3	

HYDRATION   ◇ ◇ ◇ ◇ ◇ ◇ ◇ ◇

ACTIVITY	DURATION	NOTES

MOOD	MORNING	AFTERNOON	EVENING

HOW I FELT ABOUT TODAY	ADDITIONAL NOTES

DATE_____ SLEEP_____HOURS

QUALITY OF SLEEP   ○ POOR   ○ ADEQUATE   ○ GOOD

MEAL 1	SNACKS / BEVERAGES
MEAL 2	
MEAL 3	

HYDRATION ◇ ◇ ◇ ◇ ◇ ◇ ◇ ◇

ACTIVITY	DURATION	NOTES

MOOD	MORNING	AFTERNOON	EVENING

HOW I FELT ABOUT TODAY	ADDITIONAL NOTES

DATE.. SLEEP.............HOURS

QUALITY OF SLEEP ◯ POOR   ◯ ADEQUATE   ◯ GOOD

MEAL 1	SNACKS / BEVERAGES
MEAL 2	
MEAL 3	

HYDRATION ◇ ◇ ◇ ◇ ◇ ◇ ◇ ◇

ACTIVITY	DURATION	NOTES

MOOD	MORNING	AFTERNOON	EVENING
HOW I FELT ABOUT TODAY	ADDITIONAL NOTES		

DATE_____ SLEEP_____HOURS

QUALITY OF SLEEP ○ POOR ○ ADEQUATE ○ GOOD

MEAL 1	SNACKS / BEVERAGES
MEAL 2	
MEAL 3	

HYDRATION ◇ ◇ ◇ ◇ ◇ ◇ ◇ ◇

ACTIVITY	DURATION	NOTES

MOOD	MORNING	AFTERNOON	EVENING

HOW I FELT ABOUT TODAY	ADDITIONAL NOTES

DATE.. SLEEP .... HOURS

QUALITY OF SLEEP   ○ POOR   ○ ADEQUATE   ○ GOOD

MEAL 1	SNACKS / BEVERAGES
MEAL 2	
MEAL 3	

HYDRATION   ◇ ◇ ◇ ◇ ◇ ◇ ◇ ◇

ACTIVITY	DURATION	NOTES

MOOD	MORNING	AFTERNOON	EVENING

HOW I FELT ABOUT TODAY	ADDITIONAL NOTES

DATE_____ SLEEP_____HOURS

QUALITY OF SLEEP　　○ POOR　　○ ADEQUATE　　○ GOOD

MEAL 1	SNACKS / BEVERAGES
MEAL 2	
MEAL 3	

HYDRATION　◇　◇　◇　◇　◇　◇　◇　◇

ACTIVITY	DURATION	NOTES

MOOD	MORNING	AFTERNOON	EVENING

HOW I FELT ABOUT TODAY	ADDITIONAL NOTES

DATE _____ SLEEP _____ HOURS

QUALITY OF SLEEP ○ POOR ○ ADEQUATE ○ GOOD

MEAL 1	SNACKS / BEVERAGES
MEAL 2	
MEAL 3	

HYDRATION ◇ ◇ ◇ ◇ ◇ ◇ ◇ ◇

ACTIVITY	DURATION	NOTES

MOOD	MORNING	AFTERNOON	EVENING

HOW I FELT ABOUT TODAY	ADDITIONAL NOTES

DATE... SLEEP.................HOURS

QUALITY OF SLEEP ○ POOR ○ ADEQUATE ○ GOOD

MEAL 1	SNACKS / BEVERAGES
MEAL 2	
MEAL 3	

HYDRATION ◇ ◇ ◇ ◇ ◇ ◇ ◇ ◇

ACTIVITY	DURATION	NOTES

MOOD	MORNING	AFTERNOON	EVENING

HOW I FELT ABOUT TODAY	ADDITIONAL NOTES

DATE_____ SLEEP_____HOURS

QUALITY OF SLEEP ○ POOR ○ ADEQUATE ○ GOOD

MEAL 1	SNACKS / BEVERAGES
MEAL 2	
MEAL 3	

HYDRATION ◇ ◇ ◇ ◇ ◇ ◇ ◇ ◇

ACTIVITY	DURATION	NOTES

MOOD	MORNING	AFTERNOON	EVENING

HOW I FELT ABOUT TODAY	ADDITIONAL NOTES

DATE_____ SLEEP_____HOURS

QUALITY OF SLEEP   ◯ POOR   ◯ ADEQUATE   ◯ GOOD

MEAL 1	SNACKS / BEVERAGES
MEAL 2	
MEAL 3	

HYDRATION   ◇ ◇ ◇ ◇ ◇ ◇ ◇ ◇

ACTIVITY	DURATION	NOTES

MOOD	MORNING	AFTERNOON	EVENING

HOW I FELT ABOUT TODAY	ADDITIONAL NOTES

DATE.. SLEEP............HOURS

QUALITY OF SLEEP ◯ POOR ◯ ADEQUATE ◯ GOOD

MEAL 1	SNACKS / BEVERAGES
MEAL 2	
MEAL 3	

HYDRATION ◇ ◇ ◇ ◇ ◇ ◇ ◇ ◇

ACTIVITY	DURATION	NOTES

MOOD	MORNING	AFTERNOON	EVENING

HOW I FELT ABOUT TODAY	ADDITIONAL NOTES

DATE.. SLEEP.................HOURS

QUALITY OF SLEEP   ○ POOR   ○ ADEQUATE   ○ GOOD

MEAL 1	SNACKS / BEVERAGES
MEAL 2	
MEAL 3	

HYDRATION   ◇ ◇ ◇ ◇ ◇ ◇ ◇ ◇

ACTIVITY	DURATION	NOTES

MOOD	MORNING	AFTERNOON	EVENING

HOW I FELT ABOUT TODAY	ADDITIONAL NOTES

DATE.. SLEEP............HOURS

QUALITY OF SLEEP ○ POOR ○ ADEQUATE ○ GOOD

MEAL 1	SNACKS / BEVERAGES
MEAL 2	
MEAL 3	

HYDRATION ◇ ◇ ◇ ◇ ◇ ◇ ◇ ◇

ACTIVITY	DURATION	NOTES

MOOD	MORNING	AFTERNOON	EVENING
HOW I FELT ABOUT TODAY	ADDITIONAL NOTES		

DATE_____ SLEEP_____HOURS

QUALITY OF SLEEP　　○ POOR　　○ ADEQUATE　　○ GOOD

MEAL 1	SNACKS / BEVERAGES
MEAL 2	
MEAL 3	

HYDRATION　　◇　◇　◇　◇　◇　◇　◇　◇

ACTIVITY	DURATION	NOTES

MOOD	MORNING	AFTERNOON	EVENING

HOW I FELT ABOUT TODAY	ADDITIONAL NOTES

DATE... SLEEP............HOURS

QUALITY OF SLEEP   ◯ POOR   ◯ ADEQUATE   ◯ GOOD

MEAL 1	SNACKS / BEVERAGES
MEAL 2	
MEAL 3	

HYDRATION   ◇ ◇ ◇ ◇ ◇ ◇ ◇ ◇

ACTIVITY	DURATION	NOTES

MOOD	MORNING	AFTERNOON	EVENING

HOW I FELT ABOUT TODAY	ADDITIONAL NOTES

DATE.. SLEEP............HOURS

QUALITY OF SLEEP ○ POOR ○ ADEQUATE ○ GOOD

MEAL 1	SNACKS / BEVERAGES
MEAL 2	
MEAL 3	

HYDRATION ◇ ◇ ◇ ◇ ◇ ◇ ◇ ◇

ACTIVITY	DURATION	NOTES

MOOD	MORNING	AFTERNOON	EVENING

HOW I FELT ABOUT TODAY	ADDITIONAL NOTES

DATE.. SLEEP............HOURS

QUALITY OF SLEEP   ○ POOR   ○ ADEQUATE   ○ GOOD

MEAL 1	SNACKS / BEVERAGES
MEAL 2	
MEAL 3	

HYDRATION   ◇ ◇ ◇ ◇ ◇ ◇ ◇ ◇

ACTIVITY	DURATION	NOTES

MOOD	MORNING	AFTERNOON	EVENING

HOW I FELT ABOUT TODAY	ADDITIONAL NOTES

DATE_____ SLEEP_____HOURS

QUALITY OF SLEEP   ○ POOR   ○ ADEQUATE   ○ GOOD

MEAL 1	SNACKS / BEVERAGES
MEAL 2	
MEAL 3	

HYDRATION   ◇ ◇ ◇ ◇ ◇ ◇ ◇ ◇

ACTIVITY	DURATION	NOTES

MOOD	MORNING	AFTERNOON	EVENING

HOW I FELT ABOUT TODAY	ADDITIONAL NOTES

DATE... SLEEP .... HOURS

QUALITY OF SLEEP ○ POOR ○ ADEQUATE ○ GOOD

MEAL 1	SNACKS / BEVERAGES
MEAL 2	
MEAL 3	

HYDRATION ◇ ◇ ◇ ◇ ◇ ◇ ◇ ◇

ACTIVITY	DURATION	NOTES

MOOD	MORNING	AFTERNOON	EVENING
HOW I FELT ABOUT TODAY		ADDITIONAL NOTES	

Monthly Check-In

Date: ....

Circle the level you're at in the following areas, then answer the questions that follow.

(1 = poor, 2 = needs work, 3 = okay, 4 = good, 5 = excellent)

Diet	1	2	3	4	5
Exercise	1	2	3	4	5
Sleep	1	2	3	4	5
Stress	1	2	3	4	5
Confidence	1	2	3	4	5
Energy	1	2	3	4	5

Are there any other measurements you'd like to track?

....

....

....

....

....

....

....

How do you feel about the last 30 days? Have you been successful in meeting your goals?

What are your hopes for the next 30 days? Are there new things you'd like to improve on or work toward?

What have been your biggest challenges? Strengths?

What do you feel most proud of?

DAYS
31–60

>>

DATE _____ SLEEP _____ HOURS

QUALITY OF SLEEP ⚪ POOR ⚪ ADEQUATE ⚪ GOOD

MEAL 1	SNACKS / BEVERAGES
MEAL 2	
MEAL 3	

HYDRATION ◇ ◇ ◇ ◇ ◇ ◇ ◇ ◇

ACTIVITY	DURATION	NOTES

MOOD	MORNING	AFTERNOON	EVENING

HOW I FELT ABOUT TODAY	ADDITIONAL NOTES

DATE_____ SLEEP_____HOURS

QUALITY OF SLEEP   ◯ POOR   ◯ ADEQUATE   ◯ GOOD

MEAL 1	SNACKS / BEVERAGES
MEAL 2	
MEAL 3	

HYDRATION   ◇ ◇ ◇ ◇ ◇ ◇ ◇ ◇

ACTIVITY	DURATION	NOTES

MOOD	MORNING	AFTERNOON	EVENING
HOW I FELT ABOUT TODAY	ADDITIONAL NOTES		

DATE _____ SLEEP _____ HOURS

QUALITY OF SLEEP ○ POOR ○ ADEQUATE ○ GOOD

MEAL 1	SNACKS / BEVERAGES
MEAL 2	
MEAL 3	

HYDRATION ◇ ◇ ◇ ◇ ◇ ◇ ◇ ◇

ACTIVITY	DURATION	NOTES

MOOD	MORNING	AFTERNOON	EVENING

HOW I FELT ABOUT TODAY	ADDITIONAL NOTES

DATE.. SLEEP............HOURS

QUALITY OF SLEEP ◯ POOR ◯ ADEQUATE ◯ GOOD

MEAL 1	SNACKS / BEVERAGES
MEAL 2	
MEAL 3	

HYDRATION ◇ ◇ ◇ ◇ ◇ ◇ ◇ ◇

ACTIVITY	DURATION	NOTES

MOOD	MORNING	AFTERNOON	EVENING
HOW I FELT ABOUT TODAY	**ADDITIONAL NOTES**		

DATE_____ SLEEP_____HOURS

QUALITY OF SLEEP ◯ POOR ◯ ADEQUATE ◯ GOOD

MEAL 1	SNACKS / BEVERAGES
MEAL 2	
MEAL 3	

HYDRATION ◇ ◇ ◇ ◇ ◇ ◇ ◇ ◇

ACTIVITY	DURATION	NOTES

MOOD	MORNING	AFTERNOON	EVENING

HOW I FELT ABOUT TODAY	ADDITIONAL NOTES

DATE.. SLEEP............HOURS

QUALITY OF SLEEP ○ POOR ○ ADEQUATE ○ GOOD

MEAL 1	SNACKS / BEVERAGES
MEAL 2	
MEAL 3	

HYDRATION ◇ ◇ ◇ ◇ ◇ ◇ ◇ ◇

ACTIVITY	DURATION	NOTES

MOOD	MORNING	AFTERNOON	EVENING
HOW I FELT ABOUT TODAY	ADDITIONAL NOTES		

DATE.. SLEEP............HOURS

QUALITY OF SLEEP   ◯ POOR   ◯ ADEQUATE   ◯ GOOD

MEAL 1	SNACKS / BEVERAGES
MEAL 2	
MEAL 3	

HYDRATION   ◇ ◇ ◇ ◇ ◇ ◇ ◇ ◇

ACTIVITY	DURATION	NOTES

MOOD	MORNING	AFTERNOON	EVENING

HOW I FELT ABOUT TODAY	ADDITIONAL NOTES

DATE .... SLEEP .... HOURS

QUALITY OF SLEEP   ◯ POOR   ◯ ADEQUATE   ◯ GOOD

MEAL 1	SNACKS / BEVERAGES
MEAL 2	
MEAL 3	

HYDRATION   ◇ ◇ ◇ ◇ ◇ ◇ ◇ ◇

ACTIVITY	DURATION	NOTES

MOOD	MORNING	AFTERNOON	EVENING

HOW I FELT ABOUT TODAY	ADDITIONAL NOTES

DATE _____ SLEEP _____ HOURS

QUALITY OF SLEEP ○ POOR ○ ADEQUATE ○ GOOD

MEAL 1	SNACKS / BEVERAGES
MEAL 2	
MEAL 3	

HYDRATION ◇ ◇ ◇ ◇ ◇ ◇ ◇ ◇

ACTIVITY	DURATION	NOTES

MOOD	MORNING	AFTERNOON	EVENING

HOW I FELT ABOUT TODAY	ADDITIONAL NOTES

DATE_____ SLEEP_____ HOURS

QUALITY OF SLEEP ○ POOR   ○ ADEQUATE   ○ GOOD

MEAL 1	SNACKS / BEVERAGES
MEAL 2	
MEAL 3	

HYDRATION ◇ ◇ ◇ ◇ ◇ ◇ ◇ ◇

ACTIVITY	DURATION	NOTES

MOOD	MORNING	AFTERNOON	EVENING
HOW I FELT ABOUT TODAY		ADDITIONAL NOTES	

DATE.. SLEEP.............HOURS

QUALITY OF SLEEP ○ POOR ○ ADEQUATE ○ GOOD

MEAL 1	SNACKS / BEVERAGES
MEAL 2	
MEAL 3	

HYDRATION ◇ ◇ ◇ ◇ ◇ ◇ ◇ ◇

ACTIVITY	DURATION	NOTES

MOOD	MORNING	AFTERNOON	EVENING

HOW I FELT ABOUT TODAY	ADDITIONAL NOTES

DATE... SLEEP............HOURS

QUALITY OF SLEEP　　○ POOR　　○ ADEQUATE　　○ GOOD

MEAL 1	SNACKS / BEVERAGES
MEAL 2	
MEAL 3	

HYDRATION　◇　◇　◇　◇　◇　◇　◇　◇

ACTIVITY	DURATION	NOTES

MOOD	MORNING	AFTERNOON	EVENING

HOW I FELT ABOUT TODAY	ADDITIONAL NOTES

DATE.. SLEEP............HOURS

QUALITY OF SLEEP   ◯ POOR   ◯ ADEQUATE   ◯ GOOD

MEAL 1	SNACKS / BEVERAGES
MEAL 2	
MEAL 3	

HYDRATION   ◇ ◇ ◇ ◇ ◇ ◇ ◇ ◇

ACTIVITY	DURATION	NOTES

MOOD	MORNING	AFTERNOON	EVENING

HOW I FELT ABOUT TODAY	ADDITIONAL NOTES

DATE.. SLEEP .... HOURS

QUALITY OF SLEEP ○ POOR ○ ADEQUATE ○ GOOD

MEAL 1	SNACKS / BEVERAGES
MEAL 2	
MEAL 3	

HYDRATION ◇ ◇ ◇ ◇ ◇ ◇ ◇ ◇

ACTIVITY	DURATION	NOTES

MOOD	MORNING	AFTERNOON	EVENING

HOW I FELT ABOUT TODAY	ADDITIONAL NOTES

DATE... SLEEP...............HOURS

QUALITY OF SLEEP   ○ POOR   ○ ADEQUATE   ○ GOOD

MEAL 1	SNACKS / BEVERAGES
MEAL 2	
MEAL 3	

HYDRATION   ◇ ◇ ◇ ◇ ◇ ◇ ◇ ◇

ACTIVITY	DURATION	NOTES

MOOD	MORNING	AFTERNOON	EVENING

HOW I FELT ABOUT TODAY	ADDITIONAL NOTES

DATE.. SLEEP............HOURS

QUALITY OF SLEEP   ○ POOR   ○ ADEQUATE   ○ GOOD

MEAL 1	SNACKS / BEVERAGES
MEAL 2	
MEAL 3	

HYDRATION   ◇ ◇ ◇ ◇ ◇ ◇ ◇ ◇

ACTIVITY	DURATION	NOTES

MOOD	MORNING	AFTERNOON	EVENING

HOW I FELT ABOUT TODAY	ADDITIONAL NOTES

DATE.. SLEEP............HOURS

QUALITY OF SLEEP ○ POOR ○ ADEQUATE ○ GOOD

MEAL 1	SNACKS / BEVERAGES
MEAL 2	
MEAL 3	

HYDRATION ◇ ◇ ◇ ◇ ◇ ◇ ◇ ◇

ACTIVITY	DURATION	NOTES

MOOD	MORNING	AFTERNOON	EVENING

HOW I FELT ABOUT TODAY	ADDITIONAL NOTES

DATE... SLEEP .... HOURS

QUALITY OF SLEEP   ⦿ POOR   ⦿ ADEQUATE   ⦿ GOOD

MEAL 1	SNACKS / BEVERAGES
MEAL 2	
MEAL 3	

HYDRATION   ◇   ◇   ◇   ◇   ◇   ◇   ◇   ◇

ACTIVITY	DURATION	NOTES

MOOD	MORNING	AFTERNOON	EVENING

HOW I FELT ABOUT TODAY	ADDITIONAL NOTES

DATE_____ SLEEP_____HOURS

QUALITY OF SLEEP   ○ POOR   ○ ADEQUATE   ○ GOOD

MEAL 1	SNACKS / BEVERAGES
MEAL 2	
MEAL 3	

HYDRATION ◇ ◇ ◇ ◇ ◇ ◇ ◇ ◇

ACTIVITY	DURATION	NOTES

MOOD	MORNING	AFTERNOON	EVENING

HOW I FELT ABOUT TODAY	ADDITIONAL NOTES

DATE.. SLEEP............ HOURS

QUALITY OF SLEEP   ◯ POOR   ◯ ADEQUATE   ◯ GOOD

MEAL 1	SNACKS / BEVERAGES
MEAL 2	
MEAL 3	

HYDRATION   ◇ ◇ ◇ ◇ ◇ ◇ ◇ ◇

ACTIVITY	DURATION	NOTES

MOOD	MORNING	AFTERNOON	EVENING
HOW I FELT ABOUT TODAY		ADDITIONAL NOTES	

DATE.. SLEEP............. : HOURS

QUALITY OF SLEEP ◯ POOR ◯ ADEQUATE ◯ GOOD

MEAL 1	SNACKS / BEVERAGES
MEAL 2	
MEAL 3	

HYDRATION ◇ ◇ ◇ ◇ ◇ ◇ ◇ ◇

ACTIVITY	DURATION	NOTES

MOOD	MORNING	AFTERNOON	EVENING

HOW I FELT ABOUT TODAY	ADDITIONAL NOTES

DATE.. SLEEP............HOURS

QUALITY OF SLEEP ◯ POOR ◯ ADEQUATE ◯ GOOD

MEAL 1	SNACKS / BEVERAGES
MEAL 2	
MEAL 3	

HYDRATION ◇ ◇ ◇ ◇ ◇ ◇ ◇ ◇

ACTIVITY	DURATION	NOTES

MOOD	MORNING	AFTERNOON	EVENING
HOW I FELT ABOUT TODAY		ADDITIONAL NOTES	

DATE_____ SLEEP_____HOURS

QUALITY OF SLEEP   ○ POOR   ○ ADEQUATE   ○ GOOD

MEAL 1	SNACKS / BEVERAGES
MEAL 2	
MEAL 3	

HYDRATION   ◇ ◇ ◇ ◇ ◇ ◇ ◇ ◇

ACTIVITY	DURATION	NOTES

MOOD	MORNING	AFTERNOON	EVENING

HOW I FELT ABOUT TODAY	ADDITIONAL NOTES

DATE.. SLEEP.............HOURS

QUALITY OF SLEEP   ○ POOR   ○ ADEQUATE   ○ GOOD

MEAL 1	SNACKS / BEVERAGES
MEAL 2	
MEAL 3	

HYDRATION   ◇ ◇ ◇ ◇ ◇ ◇ ◇ ◇

ACTIVITY	DURATION	NOTES

MOOD	MORNING	AFTERNOON	EVENING
HOW I FELT ABOUT TODAY	ADDITIONAL NOTES		

DATE.. SLEEP................HOURS

QUALITY OF SLEEP ○ POOR ○ ADEQUATE ○ GOOD

MEAL 1	SNACKS / BEVERAGES
MEAL 2	
MEAL 3	

HYDRATION ◇ ◇ ◇ ◇ ◇ ◇ ◇ ◇

ACTIVITY	DURATION	NOTES

MOOD	MORNING	AFTERNOON	EVENING

HOW I FELT ABOUT TODAY	ADDITIONAL NOTES

DATE... SLEEP.............HOURS

QUALITY OF SLEEP   ◯ POOR   ◯ ADEQUATE   ◯ GOOD

MEAL 1	SNACKS / BEVERAGES
MEAL 2	
MEAL 3	

HYDRATION   ◇ ◇ ◇ ◇ ◇ ◇ ◇ ◇

ACTIVITY	DURATION	NOTES

MOOD	MORNING	AFTERNOON	EVENING
HOW I FELT ABOUT TODAY		ADDITIONAL NOTES	

DATE.. SLEEP............HOURS

QUALITY OF SLEEP   ◯ POOR   ◯ ADEQUATE   ◯ GOOD

MEAL 1	SNACKS / BEVERAGES
MEAL 2	
MEAL 3	

HYDRATION   ◇   ◇   ◇   ◇   ◇   ◇   ◇   ◇

ACTIVITY	DURATION	NOTES

MOOD	MORNING	AFTERNOON	EVENING

HOW I FELT ABOUT TODAY	ADDITIONAL NOTES

DATE_____ SLEEP_____HOURS

QUALITY OF SLEEP   ◯ POOR   ◯ ADEQUATE   ◯ GOOD

MEAL 1	SNACKS / BEVERAGES
MEAL 2	
MEAL 3	

HYDRATION   ◇ ◇ ◇ ◇ ◇ ◇ ◇ ◇

ACTIVITY	DURATION	NOTES

MOOD	MORNING	AFTERNOON	EVENING

HOW I FELT ABOUT TODAY	ADDITIONAL NOTES

DATE.. SLEEP................HOURS

QUALITY OF SLEEP   ○ POOR   ○ ADEQUATE   ○ GOOD

MEAL 1	SNACKS / BEVERAGES
MEAL 2	
MEAL 3	

HYDRATION   ◇ ◇ ◇ ◇ ◇ ◇ ◇ ◇

ACTIVITY	DURATION	NOTES

MOOD	MORNING	AFTERNOON	EVENING

HOW I FELT ABOUT TODAY	ADDITIONAL NOTES

DATE.. SLEEP.................HOURS

QUALITY OF SLEEP ◯ POOR ◯ ADEQUATE ◯ GOOD

MEAL 1	SNACKS / BEVERAGES
MEAL 2	
MEAL 3	

HYDRATION ◇ ◇ ◇ ◇ ◇ ◇ ◇ ◇

ACTIVITY	DURATION	NOTES

MOOD	MORNING	AFTERNOON	EVENING

HOW I FELT ABOUT TODAY	ADDITIONAL NOTES

Monthly Check-In

Date: ....

Circle the level you're at in the following areas, then answer the questions that follow.

(1 = poor, 2 = needs work, 3 = okay, 4 = good, 5 = excellent)

Diet	1	2	3	4	5
Exercise	1	2	3	4	5
Sleep	1	2	3	4	5
Stress	1	2	3	4	5
Confidence	1	2	3	4	5
Energy	1	2	3	4	5

Are there other measurements you'd like to track?

....
....
....
....
....
....
....

How do you feel about the last 30 days? Have you been successful in meeting your goals?

....

....

....

....

....

....

What are your hopes for the next 30 days? Are there new things you'd like to improve on or work toward?

....

....

....

....

....

....

What have been your biggest challenges? Strengths?

....

....

....

....

....

....

What do you feel most proud of?

....

....

....

....

....

....

DAYS
61–90

>>>

DATE.. SLEEP.............HOURS

QUALITY OF SLEEP ◯ POOR ◯ ADEQUATE ◯ GOOD

MEAL 1	SNACKS / BEVERAGES
MEAL 2	
MEAL 3	

HYDRATION ◇ ◇ ◇ ◇ ◇ ◇ ◇ ◇

ACTIVITY	DURATION	NOTES

MOOD	MORNING	AFTERNOON	EVENING

HOW I FELT ABOUT TODAY	ADDITIONAL NOTES

DATE.. SLEEP............HOURS

QUALITY OF SLEEP ○ POOR ○ ADEQUATE ○ GOOD

MEAL 1	SNACKS / BEVERAGES
MEAL 2	
MEAL 3	

HYDRATION ◇ ◇ ◇ ◇ ◇ ◇ ◇ ◇

ACTIVITY	DURATION	NOTES

MOOD	MORNING	AFTERNOON	EVENING

HOW I FELT ABOUT TODAY	ADDITIONAL NOTES

DATE.. SLEEP................HOURS

QUALITY OF SLEEP ◯ POOR   ◯ ADEQUATE   ◯ GOOD

MEAL 1	SNACKS / BEVERAGES
MEAL 2	
MEAL 3	

HYDRATION ◇ ◇ ◇ ◇ ◇ ◇ ◇ ◇

ACTIVITY	DURATION	NOTES

MOOD	MORNING	AFTERNOON	EVENING

HOW I FELT ABOUT TODAY	ADDITIONAL NOTES

DATE.. SLEEP............HOURS

QUALITY OF SLEEP ⭘ POOR ⭘ ADEQUATE ⭘ GOOD

MEAL 1	SNACKS / BEVERAGES
MEAL 2	
MEAL 3	

HYDRATION ◇ ◇ ◇ ◇ ◇ ◇ ◇ ◇

ACTIVITY	DURATION	NOTES

MOOD	MORNING	AFTERNOON	EVENING

HOW I FELT ABOUT TODAY	ADDITIONAL NOTES

DATE.. SLEEP............HOURS

QUALITY OF SLEEP　　○ POOR　　○ ADEQUATE　　○ GOOD

MEAL 1	SNACKS / BEVERAGES
MEAL 2	
MEAL 3	

HYDRATION　　◇　◇　◇　◇　◇　◇　◇　◇

ACTIVITY	DURATION	NOTES

MOOD	MORNING	AFTERNOON	EVENING

HOW I FELT ABOUT TODAY	ADDITIONAL NOTES

DATE.. SLEEP............HOURS

QUALITY OF SLEEP   ◯ POOR   ◯ ADEQUATE   ◯ GOOD

MEAL 1	SNACKS / BEVERAGES
MEAL 2	
MEAL 3	

HYDRATION   ◇   ◇   ◇   ◇   ◇   ◇   ◇   ◇

ACTIVITY	DURATION	NOTES

MOOD	MORNING	AFTERNOON	EVENING

HOW I FELT ABOUT TODAY	ADDITIONAL NOTES

DATE.. SLEEP.............HOURS

QUALITY OF SLEEP   ○ POOR   ○ ADEQUATE   ○ GOOD

MEAL 1	SNACKS / BEVERAGES
MEAL 2	
MEAL 3	

HYDRATION   ◇ ◇ ◇ ◇ ◇ ◇ ◇ ◇

ACTIVITY	DURATION	NOTES

MOOD	MORNING	AFTERNOON	EVENING

HOW I FELT ABOUT TODAY	ADDITIONAL NOTES

DATE _____ SLEEP _____ HOURS

QUALITY OF SLEEP   ○ POOR   ○ ADEQUATE   ○ GOOD

MEAL 1	SNACKS / BEVERAGES
MEAL 2	
MEAL 3	

HYDRATION   ◇ ◇ ◇ ◇ ◇ ◇ ◇ ◇

ACTIVITY	DURATION	NOTES

MOOD	MORNING	AFTERNOON	EVENING

HOW I FELT ABOUT TODAY	ADDITIONAL NOTES

DATE.. SLEEP..............HOURS

QUALITY OF SLEEP ○ POOR ○ ADEQUATE ○ GOOD

MEAL 1	SNACKS / BEVERAGES
MEAL 2	
MEAL 3	

HYDRATION ◇ ◇ ◇ ◇ ◇ ◇ ◇ ◇

ACTIVITY	DURATION	NOTES

MOOD	MORNING	AFTERNOON	EVENING

HOW I FELT ABOUT TODAY	ADDITIONAL NOTES

DATE.. SLEEP.............HOURS

QUALITY OF SLEEP　　○ POOR　　○ ADEQUATE　　○ GOOD

MEAL 1	SNACKS / BEVERAGES
MEAL 2	
MEAL 3	

HYDRATION　◇　◇　◇　◇　◇　◇　◇　◇

ACTIVITY	DURATION	NOTES

MOOD	MORNING	AFTERNOON	EVENING

HOW I FELT ABOUT TODAY	ADDITIONAL NOTES

DATE.. SLEEP............HOURS

QUALITY OF SLEEP ◯ POOR ◯ ADEQUATE ◯ GOOD

MEAL 1	SNACKS / BEVERAGES
MEAL 2	
MEAL 3	

HYDRATION ◇ ◇ ◇ ◇ ◇ ◇ ◇ ◇

ACTIVITY	DURATION	NOTES

MOOD	MORNING	AFTERNOON	EVENING

HOW I FELT ABOUT TODAY	ADDITIONAL NOTES

DATE.. SLEEP.............HOURS

QUALITY OF SLEEP   ○ POOR   ○ ADEQUATE   ○ GOOD

MEAL 1	SNACKS / BEVERAGES
MEAL 2	
MEAL 3	

HYDRATION   ◇ ◇ ◇ ◇ ◇ ◇ ◇ ◇

ACTIVITY	DURATION	NOTES

MOOD	MORNING	AFTERNOON	EVENING

HOW I FELT ABOUT TODAY	ADDITIONAL NOTES

DATE.. SLEEP............HOURS

QUALITY OF SLEEP   ○ POOR   ○ ADEQUATE   ○ GOOD

MEAL 1	SNACKS / BEVERAGES
MEAL 2	
MEAL 3	

HYDRATION   ◇ ◇ ◇ ◇ ◇ ◇ ◇ ◇

ACTIVITY	DURATION	NOTES

MOOD	MORNING	AFTERNOON	EVENING

HOW I FELT ABOUT TODAY	ADDITIONAL NOTES

DATE .... SLEEP .... HOURS

QUALITY OF SLEEP　　○ POOR　　○ ADEQUATE　　○ GOOD

MEAL 1	SNACKS / BEVERAGES
MEAL 2	
MEAL 3	

HYDRATION　　◇　◇　◇　◇　◇　◇　◇　◇

ACTIVITY	DURATION	NOTES

MOOD	MORNING	AFTERNOON	EVENING

HOW I FELT ABOUT TODAY	ADDITIONAL NOTES

DATE_____ SLEEP_____HOURS

QUALITY OF SLEEP ○ POOR ○ ADEQUATE ○ GOOD

MEAL 1	SNACKS / BEVERAGES
MEAL 2	
MEAL 3	

HYDRATION ◇ ◇ ◇ ◇ ◇ ◇ ◇ ◇

ACTIVITY	DURATION	NOTES

MOOD	MORNING	AFTERNOON	EVENING

HOW I FELT ABOUT TODAY	ADDITIONAL NOTES

DATE.. SLEEP...............HOURS

QUALITY OF SLEEP   ◯ POOR   ◯ ADEQUATE   ◯ GOOD

MEAL 1	SNACKS / BEVERAGES
MEAL 2	
MEAL 3	

HYDRATION   ◇   ◇   ◇   ◇   ◇   ◇   ◇   ◇

ACTIVITY	DURATION	NOTES

MOOD	MORNING	AFTERNOON	EVENING

HOW I FELT ABOUT TODAY	ADDITIONAL NOTES

DATE_____ SLEEP_____ HOURS

QUALITY OF SLEEP   ○ POOR   ○ ADEQUATE   ○ GOOD

MEAL 1	SNACKS / BEVERAGES
MEAL 2	
MEAL 3	

HYDRATION   ◇ ◇ ◇ ◇ ◇ ◇ ◇ ◇

ACTIVITY	DURATION	NOTES

MOOD	MORNING	AFTERNOON	EVENING

HOW I FELT ABOUT TODAY	ADDITIONAL NOTES

DATE.. SLEEP................HOURS

QUALITY OF SLEEP ○ POOR ○ ADEQUATE ○ GOOD

MEAL 1	SNACKS / BEVERAGES
MEAL 2	
MEAL 3	

HYDRATION ◇ ◇ ◇ ◇ ◇ ◇ ◇ ◇

ACTIVITY	DURATION	NOTES

MOOD	MORNING	AFTERNOON	EVENING

HOW I FELT ABOUT TODAY	ADDITIONAL NOTES

DATE.. SLEEP.............HOURS

QUALITY OF SLEEP ◯ POOR ◯ ADEQUATE ◯ GOOD

MEAL 1	SNACKS / BEVERAGES
MEAL 2	
MEAL 3	

HYDRATION ◇ ◇ ◇ ◇ ◇ ◇ ◇ ◇

ACTIVITY	DURATION	NOTES

MOOD	MORNING	AFTERNOON	EVENING

HOW I FELT ABOUT TODAY	ADDITIONAL NOTES

DATE _____ SLEEP _____ HOURS

QUALITY OF SLEEP   ○ POOR   ○ ADEQUATE   ○ GOOD

MEAL 1	SNACKS / BEVERAGES
MEAL 2	
MEAL 3	

HYDRATION   ◇   ◇   ◇   ◇   ◇   ◇   ◇   ◇

ACTIVITY	DURATION	NOTES

MOOD	MORNING	AFTERNOON	EVENING

HOW I FELT ABOUT TODAY	ADDITIONAL NOTES

DATE.. SLEEP............HOURS

QUALITY OF SLEEP   ○ POOR   ○ ADEQUATE   ○ GOOD

MEAL 1	SNACKS / BEVERAGES
MEAL 2	
MEAL 3	

HYDRATION   ◇   ◇   ◇   ◇   ◇   ◇   ◇   ◇

ACTIVITY	DURATION	NOTES

MOOD	MORNING	AFTERNOON	EVENING

HOW I FELT ABOUT TODAY	ADDITIONAL NOTES

DATE _____ SLEEP _____ HOURS

QUALITY OF SLEEP   ○ POOR   ○ ADEQUATE   ○ GOOD

MEAL 1	SNACKS / BEVERAGES
MEAL 2	
MEAL 3	

HYDRATION   ◇ ◇ ◇ ◇ ◇ ◇ ◇ ◇

ACTIVITY	DURATION	NOTES

MOOD	MORNING	AFTERNOON	EVENING
HOW I FELT ABOUT TODAY	ADDITIONAL NOTES		

DATE.. SLEEP.................HOURS

QUALITY OF SLEEP ○ POOR ○ ADEQUATE ○ GOOD

MEAL 1	SNACKS / BEVERAGES
MEAL 2	
MEAL 3	

HYDRATION ◇ ◇ ◇ ◇ ◇ ◇ ◇ ◇

ACTIVITY	DURATION	NOTES

MOOD	MORNING	AFTERNOON	EVENING

HOW I FELT ABOUT TODAY	ADDITIONAL NOTES

DATE.. SLEEP...............HOURS

QUALITY OF SLEEP   ◯ POOR   ◯ ADEQUATE   ◯ GOOD

MEAL 1	SNACKS / BEVERAGES
MEAL 2	
MEAL 3	

HYDRATION   ◇ ◇ ◇ ◇ ◇ ◇ ◇ ◇

ACTIVITY	DURATION	NOTES

MOOD	MORNING	AFTERNOON	EVENING
HOW I FELT ABOUT TODAY	ADDITIONAL NOTES		

DATE _____ SLEEP _____ HOURS

QUALITY OF SLEEP ○ POOR ○ ADEQUATE ○ GOOD

MEAL 1	SNACKS / BEVERAGES
MEAL 2	
MEAL 3	

HYDRATION ◇ ◇ ◇ ◇ ◇ ◇ ◇ ◇

ACTIVITY	DURATION	NOTES

MOOD	MORNING	AFTERNOON	EVENING

HOW I FELT ABOUT TODAY	ADDITIONAL NOTES

DATE.. SLEEP.............HOURS

QUALITY OF SLEEP ○ POOR ○ ADEQUATE ○ GOOD

MEAL 1	SNACKS / BEVERAGES
MEAL 2	
MEAL 3	

HYDRATION ◇ ◇ ◇ ◇ ◇ ◇ ◇ ◇

ACTIVITY	DURATION	NOTES
.		

MOOD	MORNING	AFTERNOON	EVENING

HOW I FELT ABOUT TODAY	ADDITIONAL NOTES

DATE... SLEEP.............HOURS

QUALITY OF SLEEP ⭘ POOR ⭘ ADEQUATE ⭘ GOOD

MEAL 1	SNACKS / BEVERAGES
MEAL 2	
MEAL 3	

HYDRATION ◇ ◇ ◇ ◇ ◇ ◇ ◇ ◇

ACTIVITY	DURATION	NOTES

MOOD	MORNING	AFTERNOON	EVENING

HOW I FELT ABOUT TODAY	ADDITIONAL NOTES

DATE.. SLEEP............... HOURS

QUALITY OF SLEEP   ◯ POOR   ◯ ADEQUATE   ◯ GOOD

MEAL 1	SNACKS / BEVERAGES
MEAL 2	
MEAL 3	

HYDRATION   ◇   ◇   ◇   ◇   ◇   ◇   ◇   ◇

ACTIVITY	DURATION	NOTES

MOOD	MORNING	AFTERNOON	EVENING

HOW I FELT ABOUT TODAY	ADDITIONAL NOTES

DATE.. SLEEP............HOURS

QUALITY OF SLEEP ○ POOR ○ ADEQUATE ○ GOOD

MEAL 1	SNACKS / BEVERAGES
MEAL 2	
MEAL 3	

HYDRATION ◇ ◇ ◇ ◇ ◇ ◇ ◇ ◇

ACTIVITY	DURATION	NOTES

MOOD	MORNING	AFTERNOON	EVENING

HOW I FELT ABOUT TODAY	ADDITIONAL NOTES

DATE.. SLEEP............HOURS

QUALITY OF SLEEP ○ POOR ○ ADEQUATE ○ GOOD

MEAL 1	SNACKS / BEVERAGES
MEAL 2	
MEAL 3	

HYDRATION ◇ ◇ ◇ ◇ ◇ ◇ ◇ ◇

ACTIVITY	DURATION	NOTES

MOOD	MORNING	AFTERNOON	EVENING

HOW I FELT ABOUT TODAY	ADDITIONAL NOTES

Monthly Check-In

Date: ....

Circle the level you're at in the following areas, then answer the questions that follow.

(1 = poor, 2 = needs work, 3 = okay, 4 = good, 5 = excellent)

Diet	1	2	3	4	5
Exercise	1	2	3	4	5
Sleep	1	2	3	4	5
Stress	1	2	3	4	5
Confidence	1	2	3	4	5
Energy	1	2	3	4	5

Are there other measurements you'd like to track?

....

....

....

....

....

....

....

How do you feel about the last 30 days? Have you been successful in meeting your goals?

_____

_____

_____

_____

_____

What are your hopes for the future? Are there new things you'd like to improve on or work toward?

_____

_____

_____

_____

_____

What have been your biggest challenges? Strengths?

_____

_____

_____

_____

_____

What do you feel most proud of?

_____

_____

_____

_____

_____

Interior and Cover Designer: Brieanna Hattey Felschow
Art Producer: Hannah Dickerson
Editor: Rebecca Markley
Production Editor: Jax Berman
Production Manager: Holly Haydash

All illustrations used under license from The Noun Project.
All textures used under license from Shutterstock.

Paperback ISBN: 978-1-63807-486-1
R0

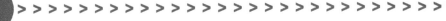